I0447684

Hair Envy
A Story of Self Perception

Dedicated to Fred Perkins

@brat Publishing

Printed by: Create Space
Editor: Alison Figueroa
Book Design & cover: Alison Figueroa
@brat Publishing
Waldorf, MD 20602
Phone 917-653-9287

Available from Amazon.com and other reatail outlets

CHAPTER I

Do You, Boo

This is the story of how I learned to love me, all of me, hair and all. Who am I, you ask? I am a regular schoolteacher born and raised in Capitol Heights, Maryland—but everybody has a story to tell. If my story helps one person, then I've done my part.

Let me start by saying that I am a black woman, who chooses to keep her hair natural. This means I decided to keep chemicals out of my hair. No, I am not one of those naturals who put down black women who are not natural. I've seen plenty of women with beautiful, flowing, healthy looking relaxed hair, which seemed to be thriving regardless of the chemical treatment. This simply isn't the case for me. I feel that a woman needs to do what works best for her. With that being said, here is my hair story.

Since I was a young girl, I remember constantly being jealous of the black girls

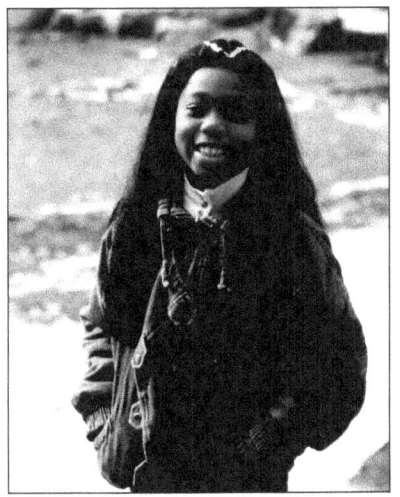
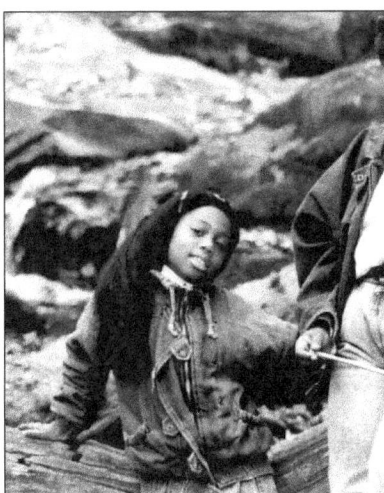

My witch hair I wore even after Halloween, just because I wanted long hair.

in my class who had what I considered pretty hair. Pretty hair to me meant wavy, curly, or long hair; but mainly long. I constantly asked the girls "what does your mom put in your hair?" I thought it must have been a magical potion that made their hair so beautiful. One day, I convinced a classmate to bring me what she used which was Pink Oil Moisturizer. She put it inside one of the black containers our parents kept a roll of film in during that time. (Now I'm telling my age.) I remember crying because it didn't make my hair curly like my friends. I couldn't understand why it didn't work. She said that was what she used, so why didn't it work? I remember being so mad at her because I assumed she lied to me.

One year, I was a witch for Halloween and the costume came with a wig. I wore the wig everywhere I went for months. My parents begged me to take it off, but I threw a fit. The funny part about the wig was it had silver streaks in it; but I didn't care. All I knew was that I had long flowing hair, like the girls I saw on the television, and you couldn't tell me anything. I just wanted anybody's hair but my own. I even remember being furious at my mom for cutting her hair. I recall looking at pictures of her when she was younger. Her hair was extremely thick and long. I wondered why I didn't inherit hair like hers and thought maybe it was because she cut her hair before I was born; so, I was mad at her too. I laugh about it now, but as a child that was no laughing matter I assure you.

I gained an obsession for craving long hair. I even went as far as to cut the hair off of one of my dolls, attach it to the end of my pony tail, and use the big balls every black girl swung in their heads during that era. You know what I'm talking

This was my mother when she had long thick hair. I wish she didn't cut it.

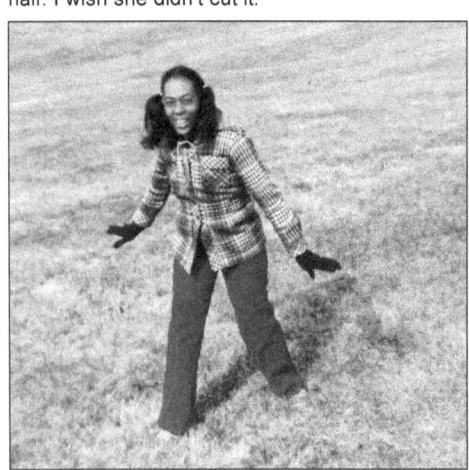

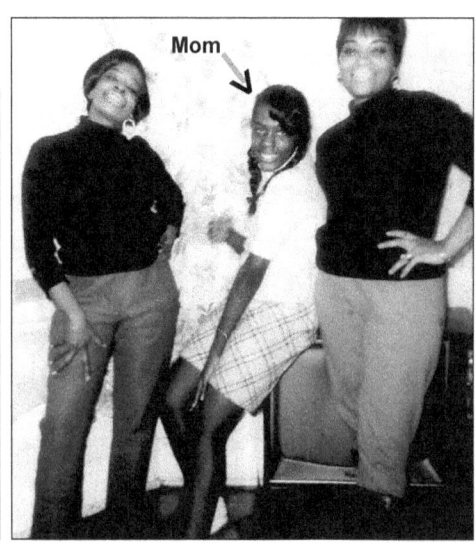
Mom

about, the ones big enough to take an eye out if you swung your head too hard. It fell off one day outside at recess as I was jumping rope. Needless to say, I was embarrassed. I covered it with my foot and when no one was looking I hurriedly picked it up and stuck it in my pocket. The sad part was I had a nice length of hair, as a matter of fact, it was longer than most of the other girls in my class. My hair was past my shoulders, but I wanted it to be long like Rudy Huxtable's from the Cosby show or Ashley's from the Fresh Prince of Bel Air.

This obsession continued into my teenage years. As a teenager, I sat in church and stared at the ladies hair sitting in the pew in front of me. I know, I know, that's bad right? I told you I had a problem. I couldn't wait until service was over so I could ask her "Who does your hair?" I thought to myself, maybe my problem was I haven't found the right stylist. My yearning for pretty hair got so out of hand I thought that every stylist in the world was out to get me. Why in the world, to this day, does stylist always cut your hair when all you asked for is a simple trim? You know what I'm talking about, but I progressed.

I can't remember how old I was when my mom began using relaxers in my hair. However, I know I don't remember a time when my hair wasn't relaxed. I used to love when my mom washed my hair and blow dry it. My hair was all blown out, huge, and crazy. I never knew what my natural hair looked like nor did I have the opportunity to see if I would even like my natural hair. Mothers don't mean any harm when they relax their daughter's hair. All they know is they want their daughter's hair to be more manageable.

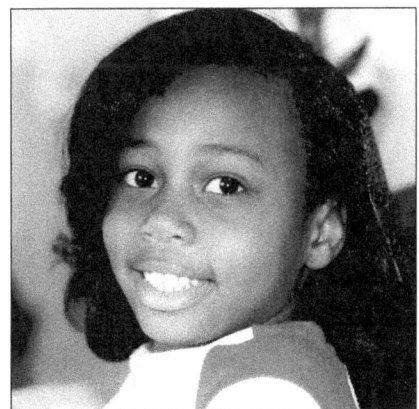 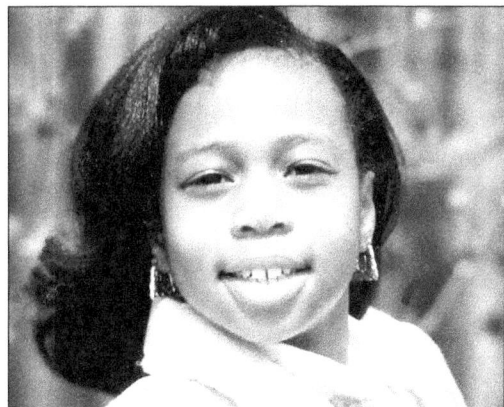

Although I had thick beautiful hair, I still wanted my hair to be as long as Rudy Huxtable's.

I had a friend who had natural hair. Her family was from Haiti and they were new to the neighborhood. Her mother didn't let her relax her hair until she went to high school, although she begged her mother every day. I remember how badly she used to get teased. I didn't want to be teased, so I was okay with a relaxer in my hair.

I never questioned getting a relaxer in my hair since it was something I received when I was a child. It became a routine to have a relaxer placed in my hair. I presumed getting relaxers were something every black woman in the world simply did. I even started putting them in by myself once I got into high school. (You think you're grown once you hit high school right?)

As I got older, I noticed my hair getting thinner and thinner each year. I didn't like this. I always looked at other girls with hair envy wishing I had what they had. Fortunate for me, extensions and sewn-in weaves became a hair fashion. Yet, this was more hair torture. If only I knew back then what I know now. Due to my painstakingly torturous hair adventures, I can now help educate other young black girls and keep them from making the same mistakes I made.

Yearbook Photo

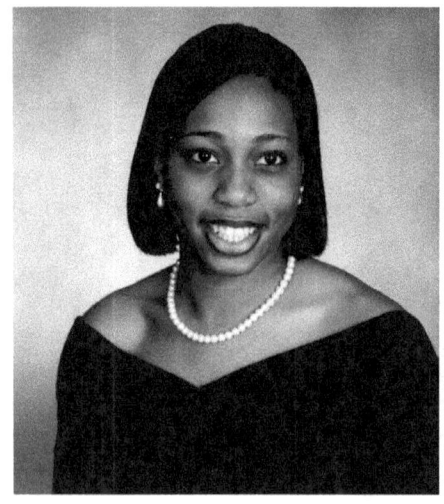

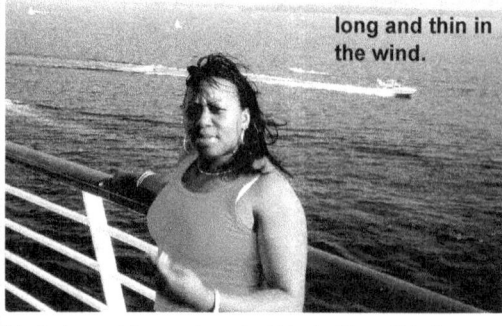

long and thin in the wind.

My hair would grow long but I hated how thin it was.

CHAPTER 2

UnNatural

One day, while standing in line at the grocery store, I heard someone ask a lady "When did you decide to go natural?" Her response was "I didn't go natural. I stopped being unnatural." She said she got the saying out of a book. I thought that was a cool response, so now I use it whenever anyone asks me that question.

When I became an elementary school teacher, I noticed all these little black girls running around with weaves and fake ponytails and it disturbed me. These were elementary school students. I felt as if, at a very young age, parents are teaching our daughters that they are not beautiful unless they add something to themselves. One girl confessed to me that she didn't feel pretty without her fake hair. This broke my heart. One of my students came to me in tears, one day, because the other girls were calling her bald headed. She explained to me that her hair was so fine because her aunt gave her a relaxer at the age of two. Funny how even a fourth grader realized there is something wrong with that. Another one of my students told me "Light skinned people look better than brown skinned people." She herself is brown, but she claimed "I am not brown! I just have a tan!" Well, to say the least, she had that tan the whole school year.

I wanted these young girls to know that they are perfect just the way God made them because He doesn't make any mistakes. But, how could I do that if I was all weaved up with a relaxer? I knew I needed to lead by example. I can remember an instance when I didn't know how to respond to a co-worker when I told her I was going to go natural. She asked "What are you trying to prove? I know you're going to straighten it sooner or later." And that was all the motivation I needed.

I recall going into my bathroom with a pair of scissors and chopping my hair away. I had no clue what I was doing, but when I was finished I had a sense of freedom.

I don't even know how to explain it. For the first time in my life. I was able to take a shower like a Caucasian woman; meaning without the use of a shower cap and my head under the water. It felt liberating to not have to worry about ruining my relaxer because water touched it. If you didn't know, water is the enemy to a relaxed sistah. You're like a slave to it:

- You hate going out if it's raining
- Don't want to go swimming, and
- Forget working out because you might sweat too much.

It sounds crazy, but it's true. I have to say I don't miss my relaxer. The main thing I don't miss is spending hours in a hair salon every other weekend to maintain it. That had to be the worse part of being relaxed for me. Now when someone asks me "Who did your hair?" I enjoy being able to say "I did."

CHAPTER 3

Fishing for Compliments

Why do we care so much about what other people think? I know it's not only me ladies; so, let's keep it real please. The main person I was concerned about when I did my "big chop" was my boyfriend. What was he going to think? God forbid he didn't like it! Luckily, I didn't have that problem. It did take some getting used to but eventually he came around. I think he was mostly shocked because this happened to come out of nowhere. I didn't discuss it with him first (that is just the type of person I am). Once I have my mind set on something, there is not much you can say to talk me out of it. I felt that if he loved me, then, he can love me with or without hair. I wasn't completely bald. I wore wigs and weaves for so long that I had about six inches of new growth by the time he saw it. I simply cut off the relaxed ends of my hair and had enough hair left over to do a flat twist out. [To achieve this look, flat twist your hair at night with a holding product then take the twist out and separate them in the morning for a crinkly look.] This was my first attempt at doing my own hair.

To my surprise, the more I practiced the better I got. I started receiving compliments at work. This surprised me because I was raised to believe that natural hair was unprofessional, but that was in the 80's. Some coworkers eventually started asking me for hair advice—me! One of my Caucasian co-workers told me she liked me in my wigs better but I didn't let it get to me. Of course I wanted people to like my hair, but it didn't make a difference to me whether they did or didn't. This was honestly the first time in my life that I wasn't worried about pleasing other people.

I simply did something for me, and I didn't care what ANYONE had to say about it. It gave me a rush of confidence because, prior to becoming natural, I had very low self-esteem. Some of my closest friends didn't know. I used to be content with simply blending into the background, but with this new, attention grabbing hair, that is now impossible. I feel that my whole personality bloomed like a flower and your actual hair forces you to come out of your shell. Strangers came up to me and began asking me questions. I've never experienced anything like it.

As time went on, I found the more confidence I portrayed, the more compliments I received. This even happened on days I knew my hair looked crazy, Trust me, I wasn't fishing for compliments, but let's be honest, we all like to hear them every once in awhile. I want approval from my family because they mean the most to me, especially my mom. She always called me "Her beautiful baby girl" and I was curious to see how she was going to react to this drastic change. My feelings would not have been destroyed if my family did not like my change but it would have been a nice added bonus if they did; you know what I mean?

When it comes to family, that's a whole different can of worms. You have to definitely be strong and hold your own around family. These are the people that know they can say whatever they want to you; no matter how insensitive it is, they

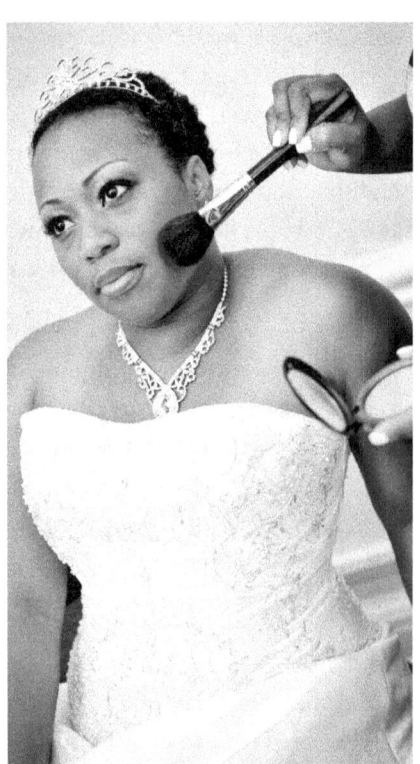 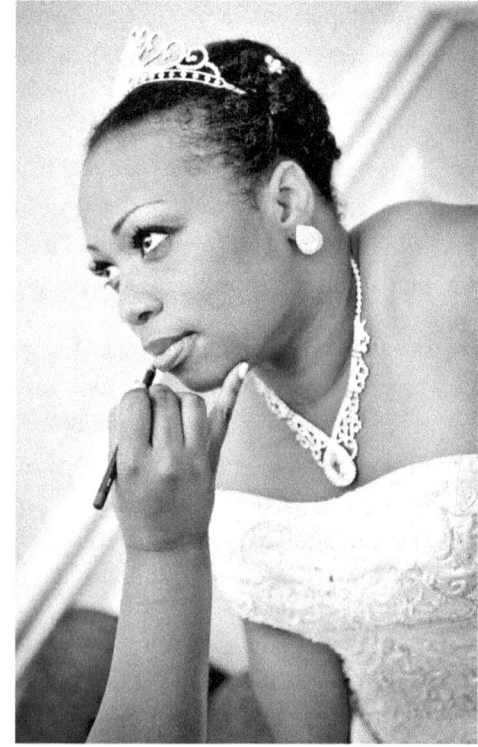

Me and my hair on my wedding day.

know they can get away with it as well. At the time of my transformation, I was contemplating getting out of teaching and getting a government job. The first thing my aunt said with genuine concern in her voice was "You know you're not getting into the government with your hair like that!" And my mom continually gave me the phone number to her friends hairdresser or anybody's hairdresser. Here lies the problem,black women refuse to take the time to learn how to take care of their own hair. Mom didn't understand that I knew my hair didn't look perfect, but I wanted to learn how to work with it on my own. I knew the more I practiced the better I would get; that was exactly what happened.

Eventually my family accepted my change and started throwing me a compliment ever so often as my hair grew. When it was time for my wedding, I was waiting for it to come up, and you know it did. "You are going to straighten your hair for the wedding, right?" Boldly I said NO and stayed firm on the issue. Every girl dreams of looking like a princess on their wedding day, and I did—an African princess. I actually did my own hair for my wedding and I felt beautiful. My husband thought I looked beautiful and that was all that mattered to me.

I never got mad at my mom & aunt for expressing their opinions. I knew they grew up during a different time where people were discriminated against because of their hair, amongst other things, so I understood their concerns. My brother-in-law, who has a light skinned wife with relaxed hair, to this day teases me often. I take it in stride and believe it is all in fun, but of course, somewhere in the back of my mind I always wonder if there is a little self-hatred going on there. Hey, that's his problem not mine. You have to grow a tough skin if you are serious about going natural because some people can and will be cruel.

CHAPTER 4

Self-Hate

This is a very controversial topic, so, I'm not going to stay on it for long. What I will say is that the majority of the negative comments I have received about my hair has been mostly from people with the same ethnicity as me. And the flip side is the majority of the compliments I have received were from EVERY other race. This is only my experience. I also noticed when I went natural, black men stopped looking my way. However, when I had relaxed hair, black men hit on me all the time. Nothing else about me changed with the exception of my hair.

My neighbor, who is a black man, told me that natural girls look like they stuck their finger in an electrical socket then proceeded to bust out laughing. I didn't find that comment funny, in fact, I found it very offensive. Blacks have been truly brainwashed to believe that what is beautiful is only the images seen in magazines and on television. I am happy to have noticed that recently more and more natural women are seen in commercials and advertisements. Although this is a great start, I would love to see us represented in sitcoms or even movie roles and not just the lady in the background sitting at a desk. I mean a leading role.

From the moment black women stepped off the boats we have been taught to be ashamed of our hair and all of our other features that make us unique. As slaves they made us wear rags on our heads to cover up our coils. We were so desperate to be accepted by Western civilization we went as far as to put bacon grease, butter, or even axel grease meant for wagon wheels, in our hair in order to straighten it. We also did other things to 'fit in' to our new forced culture. Enough is enough! It's time to embrace and love us. We are the only race whose hair grows up toward the sky. There is something to be said about that! God made us unique and that's a beautiful thing. Who are we to alter his creation? But again, as I thought before, "Do You!" These are simple reasons that encouraged me to go natural. And that's all I'm going to say about that.

CHAPTER 5

Product Junkie

Please don't think that once you go natural you don't have to do anything to your hair, in other words, you just wake up and go. Don't make me laugh; even if you are rocking a little bush hair style, you still have to take the proper steps in keeping it healthy. (And I know we all want healthy hair.) One important thing I noticed when I started my natural hair journey is that products that used to be my favorite staples when I had my relaxed hair, didn't have the same effect on my natural hair. Thus, I became a product junkie. I was on a constant search for that perfect-product that was going to give me the perfect *twist out*. The twist out is my signature style.

I'm not even going to lie to you, the search for the perfect product became very costly. A lot of these so called *natural hair care products* are overpriced, in my opinion. I found that I was getting the same or sometimes even better results from products I purchased in my local drugstore or mixtures I made myself. Unfortunately, learning that was all part of my journey and honestly, it was the fun part. Experimenting with different products and anticipating the results in the morning was all part of the learning process. Once you understand how to accomplish different styles and learn what products work best for you then you can make those products your staple products. Using your staple products all the time will allow you to spend less money.

I say products that work for you because what works for you may not work for the next person and vice versa. One co-worker asked me what products I used and I told her. She actually became infuriated with me when she tried them and they didn't work for her. Sound familiar? Everyone's hair is different and will respond differently to different products.

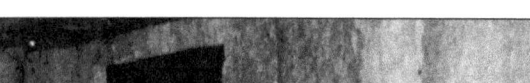

When I first went natural, I used to sit for hours and watch videos on YouTube with a notebook and pen so I can write down the name of the product the person would mention and buy them hoping they worked. I exclusively watched videos of people whose hair texture looked similar to mine. Yet to no avail, some products I tried didn't work for me. For example, every natural on YouTube raved about *Giovanni Direct Leave-In Conditioner.* I tried it expecting to be wowed and to my surprise—nothing. Everyone also raved about *Herbal Essences Hello Hydration.* I tried that; again, nothing spectacular. Then there was *Kinky Curly Knot Today.* The list of failed products is infinite but in the end I had to learn to stop listening to others and start listening to my hair.

Despite my co-worker's reaction, I didn't get mad when a product failed me—I gave them away to friends in order for them to try it. I started trying different things. I judged how well I liked it by the way it made my hair feel and that's how I found what I now call my staple products. Going natural is all about trial and error. You have to understand that you will have some bad hair days and that's okay. No, you won't get the perfect braid out or Wash & Go results every day. But let's not fake like when we had relaxed hair everyday was a perfect hair day. If it were, then you wouldn't be reading this.

Hair now is thick and healthy.

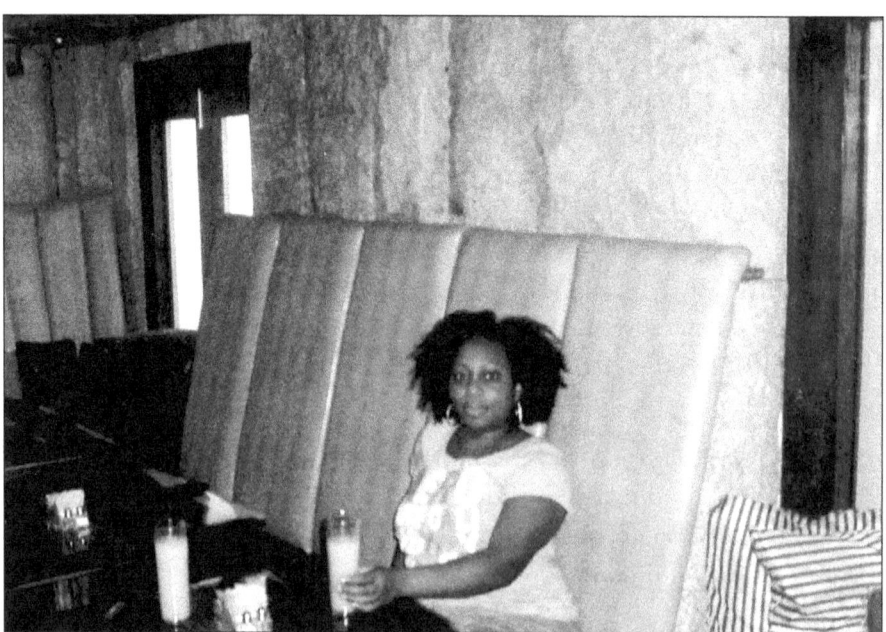

CHAPTER 6

Do Your Research

Learn how to care for your Afro textured hair

During my Hair Envy years, I used to constantly state "I'd rather have short, healthy hair than long, unhealthy hair." I repeated this motto only to make myself feel better about my hair, which didn't want to cooperate with me. I often said to myself "Just grow already!" I now realize what I didn't know before and that was my hair was short because it was unhealthy.

I used to talk about woman who kept their long hair in a bun all the time stating "What's the point of having all that hair if you're not going to do anything with it?" "If I had all that hair, I would blah, blah, blah, yackety smackety," I didn't know a thing about protective styling. I also didn't recognize that natural elements, such as wind, attack our hair on a daily basis and that hiding your ends from the wind is a defense mechanism. I was oblivious to everything.

Educate yourself and forsake listening to people and their myths. With the internet, these days, there is nothing that you can't learn about. It's been said time and time again that 'knowledge is power' and as an educator I sincerely believe that.

So let's demolish the myth that Black women's hair can't grow past their shoulders. With that being said, here's your homework assignment. Answer the following questions by doing research. You will be surprised how many videos there are about natural hair on YouTube. These are tips that I found to be interesting that I didn't know before I went natural. I feel that if I knew these things it would have saved me years of heartache. Take your time and maybe answer a question or two each day.

Let's Go…

Tip #1: What is a Protective Style?

_____
_____
_____
_____
_____
_____

Tip #2: How often should you wash your hair when it's kinky textured? What's a "Co-Wash"?

_____
_____
_____
_____
_____
_____
_____

Tip #3: What do people mean when they say, "You need to <u>seal</u> your ends?"

_____
_____
_____
_____
_____
_____

Tip #4: Moisture, or the lack thereof, is the number one reason Black women have trouble growing long hair. How can you tell if a product is a true moisturizing product? What should be the first ingredient listed?

_____
_____
_____
_____
_____

Tip #5: How come my natural hair never looks shiny even when it's moisturized?

Shine is basically the way the light reflects off your hair. The straighter your hair (Asian hair being the straightest) the shinier the hair appears to be. The reason is it's easier for the light to reflect off straighter hair. The more curly or coiled the hair is, the harder it is for light to reflect off of it. If I would have known that years ago, it would have saved me a lot of money. This is why you might have felt your hair looked shinier when it was relaxed. I hope this information keeps at least one person from searching the aisles in their local beauty supply store for another so called shine serum or oil sheen. One thing that may help you see a little difference is coconut oil. I hear a lot of naturals blog or write about this but honestly, it doesn't do anything for me.

Tip #6: A good way to protect your precious tresses is to sleep on a satin pillowcase or wear a satin cap.

Materials such as cotton can draw moisture from your hair. Even something as simple as your hair rubbing constantly against your coat or shirt all day can have damaging effects over time. This is another reason why people like to do protective styling.

Also keep in mind if you towel dry your hair after shampooing, rubbing that rough material back & forth on your fragile strands can damage it. I recommend:

- Squeezing as much water out of your hair as possible
- Use a softer material to blot the hair
- Never rub your hair back and forth over your head.

This is a reality folks, not a shampoo commercial. The way I dry my hair is, I cut an old T-shirt I don't wear anymore and use it to dry my hair. The material is very thin and soft. Sometimes I don't use anything and simply allow my hair to air-dry. The leave-in conditioner I use is thick and creamy. Once I put it in my hair, it stops the dripping. I make sure my conditioner is close by when I get out of the shower.

Tip #7: What is the correct way to detangle your hair?

_____

_____

_____

_____

_____

Tip #8: Is shedding normal?

_____

_____

_____

Tip #9: How often should you trim your ends?

_____

_____

Tip #10: What is a big chop? What is a TWA? What does it mean to transition?

_____

_____

_____

_____

_____

_____

Tip #11: Last but not least, internal health and your diet is a major factor in the health of your hair.

One of the major causes of hair loss is stress. Remember, if you don't do anything else; take care of your overall health. Exercise is known to reduce stress. And of course you know that it is important to drink water and eat healthy.

Some vitamins known for promoting healthy hair growth are zinc, iron, and biotin.

*Bonus Tip–Protein treatments can be good for the hair but too much protein can be counterproductive. If you are constantly using products that include protein, your hair can become very dry and brittle. Coconut oil is popular for being one of few oils that can actually penetrate the actual hair shaft and it is known to replace lost protein in hair. Some people are protein sensitive, so just be mindful of that. I give myself a good protein treatment at least once a month. Again, this is what has worked for me.

Sigh…

Who knew hair could be so complicated? Don't be discouraged. Afro textured hair is the most versatile hair in the world. It can be twisted and molded to hold any style. It can be worn straight, curly, or in its natural state. The options are endless once you actually take the time and learn how to work with your hair.

What's the Number One Rule?

The number one rule is to have patience! With that being said, I hope you found this informative and I wish you the best of luck reaching your healthy hair goal. Don't forget to spread the word—Black Women Can Grow Long Healthy Hair!

<u>Extra Credit Assignment</u> – What is pH balance? Why is it good to know the pH balance of your hair products, and how can you find out the pH balance of a product?

_____

_____

_____

_____

_____

CHAPTER 7

Natural Hair Stereotypes

Do I meet the criteria?

I have heard a variety of stereotypes about women who have natural hair before, during, and after my transformation. Here are a few and my responses to how untrue and ridiculous they sound.

Stereotype: All naturals want to save the earth and are tree huggers.

I am embarrassed to say that I don't even own a recycling bin.

Stereotype: Naturals love poetry.

I actually used to write poems in high school but haven't since.

Stereotype: Naturals always wear long dresses, flip flops, and big earrings.

I am a teacher; so, my husband tells me that I dress like a teacher most days—whatever that means. I do wear dresses and flip-flops in the summertime, but doesn't every girl?

Stereotype: Natural sistah's listen to Jill Scott & Erica Badu all day.

When I had relaxed hair, I adored Jill & Erica. That's just simply good taste in music. However, I also like Beyoncé, Rihanna, Chrisette Michele, old school, new school, and Gospel music. Really, I take joy in all types of music.

Stereotype: Naturals are healthy and have a strict diet of eating only organic foods.

I wish! If I could stay away from fast food chains I could fit into my favorite pair of jeans right now! Stretch pants are my new best friends. I recently decided to stop eating meat. We'll see how long that last. I'm starting to have dreams about Slim Jims.

Stereotype: Dark skin naturals are mad at the world. They hate Caucasian people, and wear black Panther T-shirts. black Power! (Feel free to throw your fist in the air.)

If I do own a shirt with a black power fist on it, it's because I think it's cute—point blank. I'm not trying to revive a movement through my fashion statements. I love being Black! I'm proud to be Black, and that's as far as it goes. I'm not dark skinned, nor light skinned either; for this reason, I think I can speak for all the beautiful darker skinned sistah's out there when I say, "Move on."

Stereotype: Naturals keep incense burning in their homes and keep a tub of Shea Butter in their pocket.

I'm a candle girl personally—vanilla scents to be exact. Yet I'm not going to lie, shea butter is the BOMB Diggity! The scent, the texture and the fact I didn't know what to do with it, deterred me from it. The discovery of vendors in Washington, DC, not too far from my home, whom whipped shea butter and blended scents in it, persuaded me to purchase the natural moisturizer. I'm in love.

The blending of shea butter gave me the inspiration to experiment and create my own mixture by adding my favorite carrier oils to it. Wait a minute, I think I should sell it— let me not get off topic. Shea butter is superb for the skin and the hair. I use it as a sealant when I do my twist outs. The results are whip lashed necks. If you decide to use it watch out now!

Stereotype: Dark skinned girls with long hair definitely have some Indian in their family. Light skinned girls with curly textured hair are mixed.

WRONG! WRONG! WRONG! The same way our skin tones comes in many different shades of brown, our hair comes in a variety of textures. This is what makes our race so beautifully unique. Don't hate! Educate yourselves people!

On the other end of the scale, a darker skinned woman, with a kinkier texture of hair, is assumed to be 100% black, when in actuality, she could be mixed. This mixture can come from her parents or grandparents because let's face it, if we really went as far back as we can possibly go, we all are mixed somewhere down the line. At the end of the day, honestly, WHO CARES?

Bottomline: Stop the stereotyping people. Gain some knowledge, because ignorance is NOT attractive. Love yourself, love other's, and the rest will fall into place. I'm done.

Peace, Love, and Hair Grease.

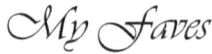

My Faves

Cheap Shampoo & Conditioner
Garnier Whole Blends Honey Treasures

Not So Cheap Shampoo & Conditioner
Hair Rules sulfate free Moisturizing Daily Cleansing Cream & Quench Ultra Rich Conditioner

Cheap Leave-In Conditioner
Herbal Essences Long Term Relationship Split End Protector

Not so Cheap Leave-In Conditioner
Curl Junkie Hibiscus and Banana Honey Butta or Curl Rehab moisturizing hair treatment strawberry ice-cream scent

(Meant to be a deep conditioner but I use it as a leave-in because it's so light.)

Styling Aid
Organic Root Stimulator Smooth and Hold Pudding

(Gave a nice *twist out* result when I first started twisting, but now I use my own mixture created by me. (See page 25.) This is pretty cheap and can be found in most drug stores or beauty supply stores. Use sparingly because a little goes a long way.

Shine or Finisher
One n' Only Moroccan Argan Oil.

(I put this on as a finisher in the morning when I take my twist out. This gives you shine and smells amazing! It's a little pricey but it's well worth it. I've tried cheaper versions but they never compare. I used to use this daily but I use it less now because my mixture gives me enough shine.)

Hair Gel
IC Fantasia Hair Polisher Styling Gel with Sparkle Lites & Aloe.

Used on my edges when I'm doing a sleek style like a bun. I also liked this product when my hair was shorter and I used to do flat twist outs. It gave me nice results.

My Mixture

I get a tub of shea butter from the beauty supply store (the type that's broken in pieces. This makes it easier to take it out of the tub).

Sit the shea in a pot of warm water to soften it. This will make mixing it easier. I melt it completely but this isn't necessary. Use the double boiler method. This can be seen on YouTube.com in case you need a visual.

Stir in 2 tablespoons each of these oils:

Coconut Oil; Jojoba Oil; Sweet Almond Oil

The coconut oil is solid but it melts to a liquid in room temperature. It will solidify and melt depending on the temperature of the room you store it in; however, this doesn't change the benefits of it.

Add a few drops of essential oil to add a pleasant fragrance to it. I use strawberry.

Stir the ingredients, then stick it in the refrigerator for about an hour to let it solidify.

My Night Time Routine

For my signature style: The Twist Out....

Step 1 I spritz my hair a few times with water using a spray bottle, just enough to dampen it. You don't want it soak and wet because it won't be dry by the morning which is a headache.

Step 2 I take my four fingers and scoop out some curl rehab and rub it all throughout my hair to moisturize, concentrating on the ends.* You can use whatever moisturizer you like.

Step 3 I take a small section of hair and put a quarter size amount of my shea butter mixture on that section of hair—sealing in the moisture. [I like this mixture because it holds and shines all in one.] I use my fingers to detangle as I twist downward. When I get to the end of the twist, I twirl it around my finger until it creates a small curl at the end.** I repeat this process until I have about 7 twist all over. The smaller you do your twist, the tighter your curls will be. I like to do medium size twist for thick wavy ringlets.

Step 4 If you have fine hair and want a little more volume and body you can put small perm rod rollers only on the ends of your twist (don't roll them all the way up to the scalp). This makes the ends a little curlier giving the hair a fuller look. I don't do this all the time. It just depends on the look I'm going for. Normally I do steps 1-3.

Step 5 Last, but not least, I cover my hair with a satin bonnet before going to sleep.

*Moisturize before styling   **Twirl to the end   The outcome

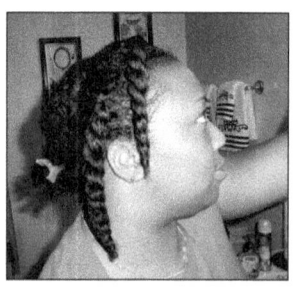
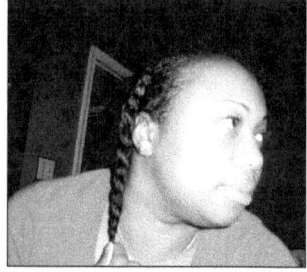
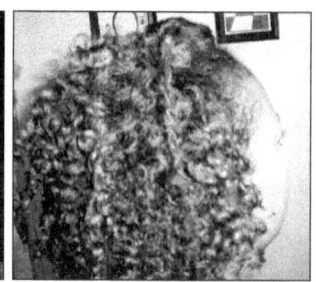

The entire process takes approximately thirty to forty minutes each night. Watching the television makes the time pass quickly. I'm used to it now. It's part of my daily routine. Again, I must stress that this is simply what has worked for me. You are welcomed to try this and I hope it helps but if it doesn't, don't be discouraged. You'll discover your regimen in due time. Eventually, as your hair gets longer your regimen may change.

Modifying....

For Step 2: You can use whatever moisturizer you choose. Keep in mind that water is the first ingredient in a true moisturizer. The *Smooth and Hold Pudding* by Organic Root Stimulator, can be used alone and you will get great results. Don't use too much because it WILL NOT be dry in the morning. You can skip *Step 3* if you use this product.

For Step 3: Some naturals like to use an oil such as Extra Virgin Olive Oil. I like using some type of butter or pomade simply because of the hold it provides. My curls last all day, unless the weather turns crazy on me. Then it's every strand for itself. My shea butter mixture seals in the moisture.

The number one cause of hair damage for Black women is dryness. NEVER put an oil based product on before moisturizing first because you will block moisture from getting into your hair. Your hair might look shiny on the outside, but inside, it's dying of thirst; and in turn, by the end of the day, it will feel dry and brittle. I know someone out there just had an "Aha" moment.

GOOD LUCK

Remember to be patient with your hair and to enjoy the journey.

Great References:

Audrey Davis-Sivasothy, *The Science of Black Hair* (Saja Publishing Company, 2011)

Ayana D. Byrd and Lori L. Tharps, *Hair Story-Untangling the Roots of Black Hair in America* (St. Martin's Griffin, NY.: St. Martin's Press, 2001).

Chris-Tia E. Donaldson, *Thank God I'm Natural-The Ultimate Guide to Caring for and Maintaining Natural Hair* (TgiNesis Press, 2008)

Bonus_ In order for you to keep track of the changes in your hair during your new transition there's a first year Natural Hair Journey journal included. By keeping a journal, you're able to keep note of the way your hair has changed throughout the transition process. In addition, keeping a natural hair journal can show you that you really are making progress in your journey, even when months later, it seems as though you aren't. Journals are also useful when you try something, LOVE the results — and then can't remember what regimen you used the next time you try to recreate the same look. If it's in your journal, you'll know exactly what you did and what products you used. My journal was my motivation to keep me going on those days that I was just ready to give up and go back to being a slave to the "creamy crack." I would look back at photos I put in it to be reminded of how far I've come. So fill it up! Don't hold nothin' back. This is the year of the new you!
Enjoy!

MY HAIR JOURNEY

Big Chop Date   or   The Day I decided to start Transitioning

_____

I felt _____
_____
_____
_____
_____

I went natural because _____
_____
_____
_____
_____
_____

Photo of Me When I was Relaxed	My First Photo Natural
PASTE HERE	**PASTE HERE**

Month One

Photo of My Hair Inspiration Person

Products I Want to Try:

```
┌─────────────────────────┐
│                         │
│                         │
│      PASTE HERE         │
│                         │
│                         │
│                         │
│                         │
│                         │
└─────────────────────────┘
```

_____
_____
_____
_____
_____
_____

My last wash day was   _____

My next wash day will be   _____

My next deep treatment day will be   _____

This Months' Length Check   inches long   _____

Products my hair liked this month	Ingredients I noticed my hair doesn't like:

My hair looked awesome today!!! This is exactly what I did:

_____

_____

_____

Month Two

Mixture I want to try & make I got from	Products I Want to Try:

My last wash day was   _____

My next wash day will be   _____

My next deep treatment day will be   _____

This Months' Length Check   inches long   _____

Products my hair liked this month	Ingredients I noticed my hair doesn't like:

My hair looked awesome today!!! This is exactly what I did:

_____

_____

_____

_____

_____

_____

Month Three

Photo of a Natural Celebrity

Products I Want to Try:

```
┌─────────────────────┐
│                     │
│                     │
│    PASTE HERE       │
│                     │
│                     │
│                     │
│                     │
│                     │
└─────────────────────┘
```

_____
_____
_____
_____
_____

My last wash day was   _____

My next wash day will be   _____

My next deep treatment day will be   _____

This Months' Length Check   inches long   _____

Products my hair liked this month	Ingredients I noticed my hair doesn't like:

My hair looked awesome today!!! This is exactly what I did:

_____
_____
_____

Month Four

Mixture I want to try & make I got from	Products I Want to Try:

My last wash day was   _____

My next wash day will be   _____

My next deep treatment day will be   _____

This Months' Length Check   inches long   _____

Products my hair liked this month	Ingredients I noticed my hair doesn't like:

My hair looked awesome today!!! This is exactly what I did:

_____
_____
_____
_____
_____
_____

Month Five

Reactions from friends & family on my new life choice	Products I Want to Try:

My last wash day was   _____

My next wash day will be   _____

My next deep treatment day will be   _____

This Months' Length Check   inches long   _____

Products my hair liked this month	Ingredients I noticed my hair doesn't like:

My hair looked awesome today!!! This is exactly what I did:

_____

_____

_____

_____

Month Six

Mixture I want to try & make I got from	Products I Want to Try:

My last wash day was   _____

My next wash day will be   _____

My next deep treatment day will be   _____

This Months' Length Check   inches long   _____

Products my hair liked this month	Ingredients I noticed my hair doesn't like:

My hair looked awesome today!!! This is exactly what I did:

_____

_____

_____

_____

_____

_____

Month Seven

Photo of Me With My Favorite Hair Style

PASTE HERE

Products I Want to Try:

_____
_____
_____
_____

My last wash day was

My next wash day will be

My next deep treatment day will be

This Months' Length Check inches long

_____

_____

_____

_____

Products my hair liked this month	Ingredients I noticed my hair doesn't like:

My hair looked awesome today!!! This is exactly what I did:

_____
_____
_____

Month Eight

What I learned about myself since I've gone natural	Products I Want to Try:

My last wash day was _____

My next wash day will be _____

My next deep treatment day will be _____

This Months' Length Check _____ inches long _____

Products my hair liked this month	Ingredients I noticed my hair doesn't like:

My hair looked awesome today!!! This is exactly what I did:

_____

_____

_____

_____

_____

_____

_____

_____

Month Nine

The best thing about being natural is	Products I want to try:

My last wash day was   _____

My next wash day will be   _____

My next deep treatment day will be   _____

This Months' Length Check   inches long   _____

Products my hair liked this month	Ingredients I noticed my hair doesn't like:

My hair looked awesome today!!! This is exactly what I did:

_____

_____

_____

_____

_____

_____

_____

_____

_____

Month Ten

What I don't miss about being relaxed is	Products I want to try:

My last wash day was _____

My next wash day will be _____

My next deep treatment day will be _____

This Months' Length Check _____ inches long _____

Products my hair liked this month	Ingredients I noticed my hair doesn't like:

My hair looked awesome today!!! This is exactly what I did:

_____

_____

_____

_____

_____

_____

_____

Month Eleven

What my significant other thinks about my natural hair is	Products I want to try:

My last wash day was   _____

My next wash day will be   _____

My next deep treatment day will be   _____

This Months' Length Check   inches long   _____

Products my hair liked this month	Ingredients I noticed my hair doesn't like:

My hair looked awesome today!!! This is exactly what I did:

_____

_____

_____

_____

_____

_____

_____

Month Twelve!!!

My Month 1 Before Photo	My Month 12 After Photo
PASTE HERE	**PASTE HERE**

My last wash day was _____

My next wash day will be _____

My next deep treatment day will be _____

This Months' Length Check   inches long _____

Products my hair liked this month	Ingredients I noticed my hair doesn't like:

My hair looked awesome today!!! This is exactly what I did:

_____

_____

_____

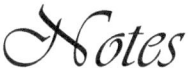 Notes

_____
_____
_____
_____
_____
_____
_____
_____
_____
_____
_____
_____
_____
_____
_____
_____
_____
_____
_____
_____
_____
_____
_____
_____
_____
_____
_____
_____
_____
_____
_____

Notes

_____
_____
_____
_____
_____
_____
_____
_____
_____
_____
_____
_____
_____
_____
_____
_____
_____
_____
_____
_____
_____
_____
_____
_____
_____
_____

Thank You for taking this journey with me and starting your own. God Bless

www.ingramcontent.com/pod-product-compliance
Lightning Source LLC
Chambersburg PA
CBHW070235290526
45789CB00004B/1628